PETE ROSE:

The Man,the Myth,the Legend-A Baseball Icon,Rise,Fall,And Unforgettable Legacy

Scott E. Adams

Pete rose

TABLE OF CONTENTS

Pete rose

INTRODUCTION

Pete Rose is a name that strikes up images of controversy, unparalleled excellence, and a lifelong passion for baseball in the chronicles of baseball history. Rose, also known as "Charlie Hustle," is a story that resonates beyond sports as he travels from the dusty fields of Cincinnati to the grandeur of the Major Leagues. We dive into Rose's unwavering quest for success, the scandal that has followed him, and the enduring legacy that validates him as a great legend of the sport in this examination of the man behind the myth. Come along as we explore the different aspects of Pete Rose's fascinating story, which is one of success, hardship, and the unwavering spirit that has irrevocably changed the diamond

CHAPTER 1: WHO IS PETE ROSE

Pete Rose, a former professional baseball player and manager who was born on April 14, 1941, is most commonly recognized for his tenure with the Cincinnati Reds. Rose was a switch-hitter who mostly played as an outfielder and infielder. He was known on the field as "Charlie Hustle" because of his unwavering work ethic. With 4,256 hits during his career, which ran from 1963 to 1986, Rose rose to the top of the Major League Baseball hits leaderboard.

Rose's legacy is clouded by dispute, though. Due to accusations that he had bet on games while managing, including some involving his team, the Cincinnati Reds, he was permanently barred from baseball in 1989. Despite his outstanding on-field accomplishments, this suspension has kept him from being eligible for acceptance into the Baseball Hall of Fame.

1.1 Early Years

Pete Rose's early years set the stage for his remarkable journey in the world of baseball. Born on April 14, 1941, in Cincinnati, Ohio, as Peter Edward Rose, he developed a passion for the sport at a young age. Raised in a blue-collar neighborhood, Rose's love for baseball blossomed on the sandlots of Cincinnati.

In his formative years, Rose's dedication and natural talent became evident. As a standout player in high school, he garnered attention for his exceptional skills on the field. Rose's relentless work ethic and determination to succeed paved the way for his entry into professional baseball.

After graduating from high school, Rose signed with the Cincinnati Reds in 1960, marking the beginning of his professional career. He quickly ascended through the minor league ranks, showcasing his versatility as both an infielder and outfielder. This swift progression foreshadowed the impact Rose would soon make on the Major Leagues.

The early chapters of Pete Rose's life in baseball were characterized by a hunger for success and an unwavering commitment to the game. Little did the world know that this ambitious young player from Cincinnati would go on to become one of the most iconic and controversial figures in the history of American sports.

1.2 Background

Pete Rose, born on April 14, 1941, in Cincinnati, Ohio, came from a working-class background. Raised in a close-knit community, Rose's early years were shaped by the blue-collar ethos of his hometown. His father, Harry Francis "Pete" Rose Sr., worked as a tool and die maker, instilling in young Pete a strong work ethic and determination.

From an early age, Rose exhibited a natural affinity for baseball. Growing up in a neighborhood where the sport was cherished, he honed his skills in sandlot games and youth leagues. Rose's competitive spirit and love for the game became apparent during his high school years at Western Hills High School in Cincinnati.

After catching the eye of scouts, Rose signed with the Cincinnati Reds in 1960, embarking on a professional career that would span over two decades. His background and upbringing grounded him in a no-nonsense approach to the game, earning him a reputation as a tenacious and hardworking player.

Beyond his baseball pursuits, Pete Rose engaged in various entrepreneurial ventures throughout his life, demonstrating a business acumen that complemented his on-field accomplishments. However, it is the indomitable spirit and gritty determination forged in the early years of his life that remain integral to understanding the man who would become known as "Charlie Hustle" – a moniker that encapsulates Pete Rose's unyielding commitment to the sport he loved.

1.3 Early Passion For Baseball

Pete Rose's early passion for baseball was a driving force that propelled him from the sandlots of Cincinnati to the grandeur of the Major Leagues. Growing up in a baseball-centric environment, Rose developed an unwavering love for the game from a very young age.

As a child, Rose found himself drawn to the rhythm of baseball games played in the streets and local parks. His initial exposure to the sport ignited a spark within him, leading to countless hours spent practicing and honing his skills. The competitive spirit that would define Rose's career emerged during informal games with friends and neighbors.

Rose's early passion wasn't merely confined to playing; he was an avid student of the game. His dedication to understanding the nuances of baseball, from strategy to technique, set him apart even in his formative years. This deep appreciation for the sport laid the foundation for the exceptional player he would later become.

It was this genuine and unbridled love for baseball that fueled Rose's journey, transforming a young enthusiast from Cincinnati into a record-breaking player and, eventually, one of the most enduring figures in the history of the sport.

1.4 Rise Through The Minor League

Pete Rose's rise through the minor leagues was marked by a combination of skill, determination, and an unyielding work ethic. After signing with the Cincinnati Reds in 1960, Rose began his professional career in the minor league system.

Rose's versatility, playing both as an infielder and outfielder, quickly caught the attention of coaches and scouts. His standout performances in the minor leagues showcased a player with an innate ability to hit, run, and contribute to the team in various capacities. Rose's relentless approach to the game, coupled with his natural talent, accelerated his ascent through the ranks.

His Minor League journey included stops with teams like the Geneva Redlegs, the Tampa Tarpons, and the Macon Peaches. At each level, Rose left an indelible mark, consistently demonstrating the skills that would later make him a Major League legend.

By 1963, Pete Rose had proven himself ready for the big stage. His successful Minor League career served as a prelude to the impactful Major League career that awaited him, ultimately solidifying his reputation as a tenacious and skilled player. Rose's rise through the minor leagues was a testament to his dedication, showcasing the early chapters of a career that would leave an enduring legacy in the world of baseball.

CHAPTER 2: THE CAREER AS A PLAYER

Pete Rose's career as a player is a storied chapter in the annals of baseball history. From his debut in 1963 to his retirement in 1986, Rose became synonymous with the Cincinnati Reds and left an indelible mark on the sport.

Pete Rose's rookie season in 1963 marked the beginning of a remarkable career that would leave an indelible mark on baseball. Here's a closer look at his rookie season and early success:

1. Debut With The Cincinnati: Pete Rose made his Major League Baseball debut with the Cincinnati Reds on April 8, 1963. At the age of 22, Rose took the field for the first time, marking the beginning of a legendary career.

2. Opponent And Venue: Rose made his debut against the Pittsburgh Pirates at Crosley Field, the former home stadium of the Cincinnati Reds.

3. Position And Versatility: He played as a second baseman in his debut, showcasing the versatility that would become a hallmark of his career as he later played

multiple positions, including outfield and third base.

4. Immediate Impact: Rose's impact was immediate, going 1-for-3 in his first game and signaling the start of a career that would be defined by consistent performance and passion for the game.

5. National League Rookie of the Year: Rose's impressive rookie season earned him the National League Rookie of the Year award, setting the stage for a career filled with accolades.

6. Impactful Batting Style: Rose's distinctive switch-hitting style added a dynamic element to the Reds' lineup. His ability to consistently put the ball in play and make things happen on the basepaths earned him the admiration of fans and teammates alike.Rose, a switch-hitter, demonstrated his ability to bat both left- and right-handed, adding a dynamic element to his play and making him a challenging matchup for opposing pitchers.

Pete Rose's debut marked the commencement of a journey that would see him become one of the most iconic figures in baseball history, ultimately leaving an indelible legacy on the Cincinnati Reds and the sport as a whole.

7. Outstanding Performance :
Rose's outstanding performance during his rookie campaign earned him the National League Rookie of the Year award.
He finished the season with a .273 batting average, 170 hits, and a league-leading 10 triples.

8. All-Star Debut: In his rookie season, Rose earned his first All-Star selection, a testament to the immediate impact he had on the league.

His All-Star debut in 1963 marked the beginning of numerous appearances in the Midsummer Classic throughout his career.

9. Setting the Stage for Greatness: Rose's rookie season laid the foundation for what would become a storied career. It showcased his work ethic, determination, and a style of play that would earn him the iconic moniker "Charlie Hustle."

Pete Rose's debut season was more than just an introduction to the Majors; it was a preview of the relentless passion and skill that would define his place in baseball history.

2.1 Cincinnati Reds Dynasty

Pete Rose played a pivotal role in the Cincinnati Reds' dynasty during the 1970s, commonly referred to as the "Big Red Machine." Here's a glimpse into Rose's contributions and the team's success during this remarkable era:

1. Integral Member of the "Big Red Machine": Rose was a cornerstone of the Reds' lineup, contributing both as an outfielder and infielder.
The team, led by manager Sparky Anderson, became a dominant force in Major League Baseball.

2. World Series Appearances: The Reds reached the World Series three times during the 1970s (1970, 1972, and 1975), with Rose playing a key role in these championship runs.
They emerged victorious in the 1975 and 1976 World Series, securing back-to-back championships.

3. 1975 World Series: The 1975 World Series against the Boston Red Sox is widely regarded as one of the greatest in history.

Rose's play, including a memorable home plate collision in Game 6, symbolized the tenacity of the Reds' lineup.

4. Consistent Offensive Performance: Rose's offensive contributions were a driving force behind the team's success. His ability to get on base, hit for average, and provide leadership in the lineup solidified his status as one of the team's most valuable players.

5. Leadership :
Rose's leadership on and off the field epitomized the "Charlie Hustle" mentality, setting the tone for the entire team.

His work ethic and determination became emblematic of the Reds' approach to the game.

Pete Rose's tenure with the Cincinnati Reds during the 1970s not only solidified his place as a baseball legend but also contributed significantly to the team's dynasty, leaving an enduring legacy in the history of the sport.

2.2. "Charlie Hustle" Persona

Pete Rose's "Charlie Hustle" persona is a legendary facet of his baseball identity, capturing the essence of his playing style and work ethic. Here's a closer look at the "Charlie Hustle" persona:

1. Relentless Work Ethic: The nickname "Charlie Hustle" was a testament to Rose's unparalleled work ethic and relentless approach to the game.
Rose was known for sprinting to first base on walks and diving headfirst into bases, showcasing his commitment to giving his all on every play.

2. All-Out Style of Play: Rose played with an intensity that resonated with fans and teammates alike. Whether at-bat, in the field, or on the basepaths, he approached

every aspect of the game with a maximum-effort mentality.

His aggressive and fearless style of play endeared him to fans and set a standard for dedication to the sport.

3. Leadership by Example: Rose's "Charlie Hustle" persona extended beyond his performance; it became a source of inspiration for teammates.

Leading by example, Rose showed that success on the field was not just about skill but also about putting in the hard work and going the extra mile.

4. Impact on Team Dynamics: Rose's energetic and hustling approach had a profound impact on team dynamics, elevating the collective spirit of the Cincinnati Reds.

His commitment to excellence influenced teammates to raise their standards and embrace a similar level of intensity.

5. Enduring Legacy: The "Charlie Hustle" moniker has become synonymous with Pete Rose's legacy. It encapsulates not just a style of play but an attitude toward the game that continues to resonate in discussions about dedication and passion in baseball.

Pete Rose's "Charlie Hustle" persona is more than a nickname; it's a symbol of the grit and determination that defined his illustrious career and left an enduring imprint on the sport of baseball.

2.3 Records And Achievements

Pete Rose, also known as "Charlie Hustle," had an impressive career with numerous records and achievements:

1. Hit King: Rose holds the record for the most career hits in Major League Baseball (MLB) history with 4,256 hits.

2. All-Star Appearances: He was selected to the All-Star Game 17 times.
Three Batting Titles: Rose won three National League batting titles during his career.

3. World Series Championships: Rose won three World Series championships, twice with the Cincinnati Reds (1975, 1976) and once with the Philadelphia Phillies (1980).

4. Most Games Played: He played in 3,562 games, setting an MLB record for the most games played by a position player.

5. Versatility: Rose played multiple positions, including outfield, infield, and first base, showcasing his versatility on the field.

6. MVP Awards: He won the National League MVP award in 1973.
Hit Streak: Rose had a 44-game hit streak in 1978, the second-longest in MLB history.

7. Silver Slugger: He was awarded the Silver Slugger Award twice in recognition of his offensive contributions as an outfielder.

Despite these achievements, Rose's legacy is complicated by his ban from baseball due to allegations of gambling on games, including his team, which led to his ineligibility for the Baseball Hall of Fame

2.4. Legacy And Impact

Pete Rose's legacy in baseball is a mix of outstanding achievements on the field and controversy off the field.

Positive Impact:

1. Hit King: Rose's record for the most career hits in MLB history (4,256) remains

a remarkable achievement, showcasing his consistency and longevity.

2. Versatility: His ability to play multiple positions demonstrated versatility and dedication to his team's success.

3. Competitive Spirit: Known for his relentless work ethic and "Charlie Hustle" mentality, Rose became a symbol of determination and competitiveness.

4. Championships: Winning three World Series championships contributed to his positive impact on the teams he played for.

2.5 Controversies

1. Banned from Baseball: Rose's ban from baseball in 1989 due to gambling on games, including his team, had a profound impact on his legacy. This ban extends to eligibility for the Baseball Hall of Fame.

2. Impact on Integrity: The gambling scandal tarnished the perceived integrity of the game and had broader implications for how players, especially those in leadership positions, were viewed about the sport's rules.

3. Ongoing Debate: The debate over whether Rose should be reinstated and

allowed into the Hall of Fame continues to be a topic of discussion among baseball enthusiasts.

4. Legacy in Popular Culture: Rose's story is often used as a cautionary tale about the consequences of actions that jeopardize the integrity of the game.

In summary, Pete Rose's legacy is a complex mix of extraordinary achievements on the field and controversies off the field, making him a figure with a lasting impact on the history and discussions surrounding baseball. Pete Rose's player years are a testament to his unparalleled dedication, leaving an enduring legacy that transcends statistics and controversies, making him one of baseball's most iconic and debated figures.

CHAPTER 3: RECORD-BREAKING ETHICS

Pete Rose's most significant record-breaking achievement is his status as the "Hit King." He holds the all-time Major League Baseball record for the most career hits, accumulating a total of 4,256 hits over his illustrious career. This record surpasses the previous mark held by Ty Cobb and stands as a testament to Rose's exceptional consistency and longevity as a hitter. His record-breaking achievement in hits is a defining aspect of his legacy in the world of baseball.

Pete Rose's achievement as the "Hit King" is a testament to his remarkable career in Major League Baseball (MLB). With a total of 4,256 hits, Rose surpassed the previous record held by Ty Cobb. This accomplishment reflects Rose's consistency, durability, and exceptional skill as a hitter. The title "Hit King" highlights his ability to make contact with the ball consistently over the course of his career, solidifying his place in baseball history. Despite the controversies surrounding his later years, Rose's record as the Hit King remains one of the most enduring and significant achievements in the sport.

3.1. The Manager

Pete Rose also had a managerial career in addition to his playing days. He managed the Cincinnati Reds from 1984 to 1989. Under his management, the Reds had notable successes, including winning the 1986 National League (NL) pennant. However, Rose's managerial career was overshadowed by the gambling controversy, leading to his ban from baseball in 1989. Despite their successes on the field, his managerial legacy is intertwined with the controversies that marked the later stages of his career.

3.2. Transition To Coaching

After his playing career, Pete Rose transitioned to coaching and managing in baseball. He became the player-manager for the Cincinnati Reds in 1984. This dual role allowed him to continue playing while also taking on managerial responsibilities. Rose's transition to coaching demonstrated his continued passion for the game and his desire to contribute to the success of his team in a leadership capacity. While his managing career had successes, including leading the Reds to the 1986 National League pennant, it was ultimately marred by his ban from baseball in 1989 due to allegations of gambling, impacting his coaching legacy.

Pete Rose's transition to coaching and managing unfolded as follows:

1. Player-Manager Appointment: In August 1984, Rose was named the player-manager of the Cincinnati Reds, succeeding Vern Rapp. This move allowed Rose to continue playing while taking on managerial responsibilities.

Immediate Impact: Rose's influence was felt immediately as the team's performance improved under his leadership. His hands-on approach and deep understanding of the game resonated with the players.

2. 1985 Season: In his first full season as player-manager in 1985, the Reds finished second in the National League West with a record of 89-72, a marked improvement from the previous year.

3. 1986 Pennant Run: The pinnacle of Rose's managerial career came in 1986 when he led the Reds to the National League pennant. They faced the Boston

Red Sox in the World Series but lost in a memorable seven-game matchup.

4. Player-Manager Challenges: Juggling the dual role of player and manager presented challenges, and there were occasional tensions with the front office over personnel decisions.

5. 1987 Suspension: Rose received a 30-day suspension in 1987 for pushing an umpire during an argument. This incident underscored the intensity of Rose's approach to the game.

6. Banning from Baseball: In 1989, Rose's managerial career came to an abrupt end when he agreed to a permanent ban from baseball. This followed an investigation into his gambling activities, including allegations of betting on games involving his team.

3.3. Legacy Impact

The ban had a profound impact on Rose's legacy as a manager, overshadowing the successes and positive aspects of his tenure.

Pete Rose's transition to coaching and managing showcased both successes and challenges, but ultimately, the controversies surrounding his gambling activities cast a long shadow over this phase of his career.

3.4. Managing Role

Rose's transition to coaching and managing in baseball was a notable phase in his post-playing career. Here are some additional details:

1. Player-Manager Role: Rose took on the role of player-manager for the Cincinnati Reds in August 1984. This unique position allowed him to continue playing while

also being responsible for managerial decisions.

2. Leadership Style: Known for his intense work ethic and competitive nature as a player, Rose brought a similar approach to his managerial duties. He was hands-on and had a keen understanding of the game.

3. 1985 Season Success: In 1985, Rose guided the Reds to a second-place finish in the National League West. This early success suggested promise for his managerial career.

4. 1986 National League Pennant: One of the highlights of Rose's managerial career was leading the Reds to the National League pennant in 1986. However, they lost to the Boston Red Sox in the World Series.

5. Managerial Challenges: Despite on-field success, Rose faced challenges off the field, including controversies and clashes with team management. The controversies were a precursor to more significant issues that would later impact his managerial legacy.

6. Banned from Baseball: In 1989, Rose was banned from baseball due to allegations of gambling on games, including his team. This ban ended his managerial career and raised questions about his overall legacy in the sport.

7. Post-Ban Impact: After the ban, Rose has remained a controversial figure, and his exclusion from the Baseball Hall of Fame continues to be a topic of debate. Pete Rose's transition to coaching and managing showcased his commitment to the game, but the later controversies significantly shaped the narrative of this phase in his career.

CHAPTER 4: CINCINNATI REDS AND BEYOND

Following his playing and overseeing vocation with the Cincinnati Reds, Pete Rose's association in baseball reached out past the Reds in different ways:

1. Post-Reds Playing Profession: In the wake of leaving the Reds, Rose played for the Montreal Exhibitions in 1984 and afterward completed his playing profession with the Cincinnati Reds in 1986.

2. Montreal Exhibitions (1984): Rose played for the Montreal Exhibitions in 1984 in the wake of leaving the Reds. Be that as it may, his experience with the Exhibitions was somewhat concise.

3. Cincinnati Reds (1984-1986): Rose got back to the Cincinnati Reds in 1984, denoting the finish of his playing vocation with the group wherein he had accomplished notable status. He played with the Reds until 1986.

4. Dealing with the Reds: Despite his restriction from baseball, Rose's

administrative profession wasn't altogether bound to the Reds. He dealt with the group until his boycott in 1989.

5. Later Administrative Spells: After his boycott, Rose endeavored to rebound in baseball. He dealt with the Cincinnati Reds in 1989 and the piece of the 1989 season.

6. Collection of Memoirs and Books: Rose composed a few books, including his collection of memoirs. These works gave bits of knowledge into his vocation, contentions, and points of view on baseball.

7. Public Appearances: Rose stayed an individual of note, showing up at games, signature signings, and other public discussions.

8.Legitimate Issues: Notwithstanding baseball exercises, Rose confronted legitimate issues, including tax avoidance charges, which brought about a five-month jail sentence in 1990.

9.Corridor of Distinction Qualification: Rose's restriction from baseball has forestalled his enlistment into the Baseball

Corridor of Popularity, despite his exceptional playing vocation.

10. Proceeded with Discussion: The discussion over Rose's boycott and Lobby of Notoriety qualification keeps on being a subject of conversation among baseball fans and specialists.

Pete Rose's post-Reds profession is set apart by a mix of proceeded with contributions to the baseball world, lawful difficulties, and continuous contentions connected with his restriction from the game.

4.1. Broadcasting

Rose wandered into broadcasting, giving, discourse for both TV and radio. His understanding and information on the game made him a sought-after investigators

Pete Rose had an outstanding profession as a baseball telecaster, giving examination and discourse on the game. His bits of knowledge and profound comprehension of the game made him a sought-after expert. A few central issues about Rose's communicating vocation include:

1. TV and Radio: Rose added to both TV and radio stations, sharing his viewpoint on games, players, and vital parts of baseball.

2. Insightful Methodology: Known for his logical methodology, Rose drew on his broad experience as a player and chief to give important bits of knowledge about the elements of the game.

3. Game Analysis: Rose frequently filled in as a variety of pundits during live game transmissions, offering critiques on plays, procedures, and player exhibitions.

4. Studio Investigation: Notwithstanding live game critique, Rose showed up in studio settings, separating key minutes, exchanges, and advancements in the realm of baseball.

5. Media Presence: Rose's media presence reached out past communicating, with interviews, board conversations, and appearances on different games-related programs.

6. Association with Fans: His immediate and authentic style resounded with fans, and he became known for giving clear and unfiltered discourse.

While Rose's communicating profession added one more aspect to his commitment to baseball, his restriction from the game in 1989 restricted his authority contribution in any MLB-associated limit, including broadcasting. Regardless of this, he stayed a conspicuous figure in the baseball local area.

4.2 Personal History And Books

Pete Rose wrote a few, including a self-portrayal, giving bits of knowledge about his life, profession, and the discussions encompassing him. A few outstanding books include:

1. "Pete Rose: My Story" (1989): This self-portrayal, co-composed with Roger Kahn, digs into Rose's life and profession, chronicling his excursion from a youthful baseball lover to becoming one of the game's record-breaking greats. It additionally addresses the betting claims that prompted his restriction from baseball.

2. "My Jail Without Bars" (2004): In this book, Rose considers his life, remembering his time in jail for tax avoidance. He examines his connections,

his encounters in jail, and the effect of his restriction from baseball.

3. "Pete Rose: An American Issue" (1992): Composed by Kostya Kennedy, this book gives an inside-and-out investigation of Rose's life and the debates encompassing him, looking at the intricacies of his heritage and its effect on the game.

4. "Hustle: The Legend, Life, and Lies of Pete Rose" (1992): Michael Sokolove's book digs into Rose's character, looking at the fantasy of his hard-working attitude

and investigating the intricacies of his vocation, both on and off the field.

5. "Pete Rose: Baseball's Charlie Hustle" (1985): Composed by Milton Gross, this life story conceals Rose's playing vocation to the mid-1980s, offering experiences into his playing style and way of dealing with the game.

These books give alternate points of view on Pete Rose's life and profession, offering perusers a more profound comprehension of the difficulties, triumphs, and discussions that characterized his excursion all through baseball.

4.3. Discussion

Pete Rose's discussion fundamentally rotates around his relationship with betting and resulting expulsion from baseball. Here are key insights regarding the debate:

1. Betting Charges: In 1989, Significant Association Baseball (MLB) explored Rose for betting exercises. The examination uncovered that Rose had wagered on ball games, including those including the Cincinnati Reds, the group he made due.

2. Consent to Expulsion: Instead of challenging the claims, Rose agreed with MLB Magistrate A. Bartlett Giamatti on August 24, 1989. In the understanding, Rose acknowledged a long-lasting restriction from baseball yet didn't expressly concede or deny the betting charges.

3. Ineligibility for Lobby of Distinction: Because of the boycott, Pete Rose became ineligible for acceptance into the Baseball Corridor of Distinction. Despite his noteworthy playing profession and being the record-breaking hits pioneer, his

boycott has kept him out of the Corridor of Acclaim.

4. Demands for Restoration: Throughout the long term, Rose has made different solicitations for reestablishment into baseball, wanting to work in the game and be considered for the Corridor of Acclaim. Notwithstanding, these solicitations have been reliably denied by MLB.

5. Legitimate Ramifications: Rose's contribution to betting likewise prompted lawful difficulties. While the concurrence with MLB zeroed in on his restriction from baseball, he confronted separate

lawful difficulties, remembering a jail sentence for tax avoidance in 1990.

6. Inheritance and Discussion: The discussion encompassing Rose's expulsion lastingly affects his heritage. There is continuous discussion among baseball fans, players, and authorities about whether he ought to be restored and permitted passage into the Corridor of Popularity.

The Pete Rose discussion remains quite possibly one of the most huge and discussed issues throughout the entire existence of baseball, bringing up issues about the connection between the game

and betting, as well as the ramifications
for those engaged with such exercises

4.4 Betting Claims

Pete Rose's betting claims date back to the
last part of the 1980s and are a focal piece
of the contention encompassing his
vocation. Here are the central issues
regarding the betting claims:
Investigation: In 1989, Significant
Association Baseball (MLB) started an
examination concerning Pete Rose's
betting exercises. The examination zeroed
in on Rose's supposed wagers on ball

games, including those including the Cincinnati Reds, the group he made due. Wagering on His Group: The most serious part of the charges was that Rose had supposedly put down wagers on games including the Cincinnati Reds, the group he was overseeing at that point. This raised worries about the respectability of the game.

1. Concurrence with MLB: Rather than challenging the claims, Pete Rose agreed with MLB Chief A. Bartlett Giamatti on August 24, 1989. In this understanding, Rose acknowledged an extremely durable restriction from baseball, however, he

didn't expressly confess to or deny the betting charges.

2. Subtleties of Wagers: The examination uncovered that Rose had put down wagers with different bookmakers, remembering for individual games. The wagers remembered bets for his group, which disregarded MLB's principles and raised moral worries.

3. Influence on Inheritance: The betting charges and resulting restrictions from baseball significantly affected Pete Rose's heritage. Regardless of being perhaps one of the best hitters throughout the entire

existence of the game, the contention has created a shaded area over his profession.

4. Restoration Solicitations: Throughout the long term, Rose has made a few ineffective solicitations for reestablishment into baseball. His expulsion has kept him from partaking in true MLB exercises, making due, or being considered for enlistment into the Baseball Lobby of Distinction.

The betting charges and Rose's restriction from baseball keep on being huge subjects of conversation and discussion inside the baseball local area.

4.5. Examinations

Pete Rose, a previous Significant Association Baseball player, was restricted for life in 1989 for wagering on games, including his group, the Cincinnati Reds. The examination found proof supporting these claims, prompting his rejection from the Lobby of Popularity. The discussion remains a critical part of baseball history.

4.6. Pete Rose Fall

Pete Rose's expulsion from baseball happened in 1989 and is a consequence of his relationship with betting. Here are key insights concerning his expulsion:

1. Examination and Discoveries: In 1989, Significant Association Baseball (MLB) directed an examination concerning Pete Rose's betting exercises. The examination uncovered that Rose had wagered on ball games, including those including the Cincinnati Reds, the group he made due.

2. Concurrence with MLB: Instead of challenging the claims, Pete Rose went into a concurrence with MLB Magistrate A. Bartlett Giamatti on August 24, 1989. In this understanding, Rose acknowledged

a super durable restriction from baseball. The understanding did exclude an admission or denial of the gambling charges.

3. Purposes behind Expulsion: The boycott was a consequence of Rose's infringement of Rule 21(d), which disallows any player, umpire, or club or association official from wagering on the result of ball games. Wagering in his group raised critical worries about the uprightness of the game.

4. Lobby of Distinction Ineligibility: As an outcome of the boycott, Rose became ineligible for enlistment into the Baseball

Lobby of Notoriety. Despite his exceptional playing vocation and being the record-breaking hits pioneer, he remains prohibited from the Corridor of Acclaim.

5. Restoration Solicitations: Throughout the long term, Pete Rose has made numerous solicitations for reestablishment into baseball. Nonetheless, these solicitations have been reliably denied by MLB, and he has not been permitted to take part in true association exercises.

6. Legitimate Ramifications: While the concurrence with MLB zeroed in on Rose's restriction from baseball, he

likewise confronted separate legitimate issues, incorporating a jail sentence in 1990 for tax avoidance.

Pete Rose's expulsion from baseball remains quite possibly the most huge and questionable occasion throughout the entire existence of the game, starting continuous conversations about pardoning, reclamation, and the connection between baseball and betting.

CHAPTER 5: LEGAL BATTLES

Pete Rose participated in an extensive fight in court following his restriction from baseball. Notwithstanding confessing to wagering on games, he at first denied betting on his own group. Throughout the long term, he looked for reestablishment, however MLB kept up with its boycott. Rose recorded numerous requests, however starting around my last information update in January 2022, he had not been reestablished, and the boycott stayed essentially. Official procedures and conversations around his boycott might have advanced from that point forward.

Pete Rose's fight in court unfurled as an outcome of his restriction from Significant Association Baseball (MLB) in 1989 because of claims of wagering on ball games, including those including his own group, the Cincinnati Reds. Here is a nitty gritty outline of the vital occasions in his legitimate adventure:

1. Restricting from Baseball (1989): MLB's examination, drove by legal advisor John Dowd, found proof

supporting Rose's association in wagering on games. In August 1989, then, at that point Official Bart Giamatti reported Rose's lifetime restriction from baseball. The boycott implied Rose was ineligible for acceptance into the Corridor of Notoriety.

2. Confirmation of Wagering (2004): In his 2004 collection of memoirs, "My Jail Without Bars," Rose confessed to wagering on baseball, including Reds games, yet he kept on denying wagering against his group. This confirmation, while a critical turn of events, didn't bring about his restoration.

3. Restoration Applications: Pete Rose applied for reestablishment to MLB on numerous events. His most memorable conventional solicitation in 1992 was dismissed by Official Fay Vincent. Ensuing officials, including Bud Selig, likewise maintained the boycott.

4. Lobby of Popularity Qualification: Rose's boycott reached out to Corridor of Popularity qualification. Notwithstanding his noteworthy vocation accomplishments, including being MLB's unequaled hits pioneer, he remained prohibited from thought for the Lobby of Popularity.

5. Lawful Difficulties: Rose sought after lawful roads to challenge the boycott. In 1990, he documented a criticism claim against John Dowd, which was subsequently settled. Nonetheless, lawful endeavors to upset the boycott demonstrated ineffective.

6. Public Mission: Throughout the long term, Rose took part in a public mission looking for reestablishment. He offered conciliatory sentiments for his activities and contended that he had served a sufficiently long punishment. In spite of

public compassion and backing, MLB kept up with its position.

7. Current Status: Starting around my last information update in January 2022, Pete Rose had not been reestablished, and the boycott stayed as a result. His fight in court highlighted the difficulties related with upsetting a lifetime restriction from elite athletics.

5.1 Reclamation Endeavor

Pete Rose has made a few endeavors at reclamation throughout the long term, looking for a way to reestablishment into Significant Association Baseball (MLB) and the potential chance to be considered for enlistment into the Lobby of Popularity. Here are a few parts of his reclamation endeavors:

1. Affirmation and Expression of remorse (2004): In his 2004 life account, "My Jail Without Bars," Rose confessed to wagering on baseball, including games including his own group. He put out a general acknowledgment for his activities, recognizing the mix-ups he had made.

2. Reestablishment Petitions: Rose officially applied for reestablishment to MLB on numerous events. These

solicitations were submitted to magistrates like Bud Selig, yet they were reliably denied. MLB kept up with its position on maintaining the lifetime boycott.

3. Advertising Endeavors: Rose participated in advertising endeavors to work on his picture and gather support for restoration. He took part in occasions, signature signings, and meetings, underscoring regret for his past activities and communicating a longing briefly possibility.

4. Lobby of Notoriety Thought: Rose's ineligibility for the Lobby of Popularity

has been a focal piece of his reclamation mission. He and his allies have contended that his on-field achievements, including being the record-breaking hits pioneer, ought to be independent from his off-field offenses.

5. Local area Commitment: Rose has been associated with different local area and noble cause exercises, expecting to exhibit his obligation to positive commitments past the baseball field.

In spite of these endeavors, as of January 2022, Rose had not been reestablished into MLB, and his Lobby of Acclaim qualification stayed unaltered.

The association has been reliable in its choice to maintain the lifetime boycott

5.2 Battle For Reestablishment

Pete Rose's battle for restoration into Significant Association Baseball (MLB) has been described by a progression of endeavors, challenges, and constant refusals. Here is a more intensive glance at the critical parts of his mission for restoration:

1. Formal Reestablishment Solicitations: Following his boycott in 1989, Rose

submitted conventional solicitations for restoration to MLB officials. Regardless of communicating regret and a longing to get back to the game, these solicitations were reliably denied.

2. Officials' Choices: Magistrates, for example, Fay Vincent and Bud Selig maintained the boycott, underlining the seriousness of Rose's activities and the need to keep up with the honesty of the game. The agreement inside MLB has been to keep up with the lifetime boycott as an obstruction against betting related infractions.

Requests and Legitimate Difficulties: Rose sought after legitimate roads to challenge the boycott, including documenting a criticism claim against John Dowd, the examiner who gathered the proof prompting the boycott. Nonetheless, these lawful endeavors didn't bring about the upsetting of the boycott.

3. Confirmation of Wagering (2004): In his 2004 collection of memoirs, Rose owned up to wagering on baseball, including games including the Cincinnati Reds. While this confirmation might have added straightforwardness to his activities,

it didn't prompt an adjustment of his boycott status.

4. Open acknowledgments : Rose participated in advertising endeavors to reconstruct his picture, saying 'sorry' for his errors and communicating lament for the effect on the game. Notwithstanding these endeavors, MLB kept up with its situation on the boycott.

5. Lobby of Distinction Ineligibility: Rose's ineligibility for the Corridor of Notoriety has been a critical obstacle as he continued looking for restoration. The Baseball Journalists' Relationship of

America has been steady in not considering people on MLB's forever ineligible rundown, which incorporates Rose.

6. Continuous Conversations: The subject of Pete Rose's restoration has occasionally reemerged, starting conversations inside the baseball local area and among fans. Be that as it may, starting around my last information update in January 2022, MLB had not switched its choice, and Rose stayed prohibited from the game.

Pete Rose's battle for restoration highlights the intricacies encompassing issues of respectability and the results of abusing baseball's standards against betting.

5.3 Legitimate Difficulties

Pete Rose confronted legitimate moves basically in his endeavors to challenge the lifetime boycott forced by Significant Association Baseball (MLB). Here are a few critical parts of the legitimate difficulties he experienced:

1. Slander Claim (1990): In 1990, Rose documented a maligning claim against John Dowd, the examiner who gathered the proof prompting his boycott. The claim affirmed that Dowd had offered

bogus expressions about Rose's betting exercises. The case was subsequently privately addressed any remaining issues, with Dowd recognizing that he didn't have proof that Rose bet against the Reds.

2. Reestablishment Requests: Rose submitted conventional solicitations for reestablishment to MLB magistrates, including Fay Vincent and Bud Selig, trying to upset the boycott. These requests depended on different grounds, including articulations of regret and the contention that he had served an adequate punishment. In any case, all endeavors at reestablishment were denied.

3. Lawful and Advertising Techniques: Rose utilized lawful techniques and participated in advertising endeavors to communicate his perspective for reestablishment. His legitimate group investigated roads to challenge the boycott, yet MLB's position stayed undaunted.

4. Lobby of Distinction Ineligibility: Rose's ineligibility for the Baseball Corridor of Acclaim because of his boycott provoked conversations about whether he ought to be thought about independently from his off-field activities.

Be that as it may, the qualification rules have not been modified, and Rose stays ineligible for Lobby of Acclaim enlistment.

5. Progressing Endeavors: Notwithstanding confronting rehashed lawful difficulties, Rose kept on communicating a craving for reestablishment. His lawful group investigated various points, remembering contentions about changes for the baseball scene and the advancing position on betting in sports.

6. MLB's Honesty and Discouragement:
One of the focal contentions against restoring Rose has been MLB's obligation to keeping up with the trustworthiness of the game and discouraging players and authorities from taking part in betting exercises that could think twice about sport

Anyway the qualification rule has not been modified and rose stays prohibited

CHAPTER 6: PUBLIC OPINION

Public opinion on Pete Rose is varied and often depends on individual perspectives within the baseball community and among fans. Here are some key points that capture the range of opinions:

1. Supporters: Some fans and members of the baseball community express empathy for Pete Rose, emphasizing his exceptional on-field achievements, including being MLB's all-time hits leader. Supporters often argue that his ban should be reconsidered, especially in light of his admissions of betting on games.

2. Critics: On the other hand, some critics emphasize the gravity of Rose's actions, particularly the allegations of betting on games, including those involving his team. Critics argue that upholding the ban is essential to maintaining the integrity of the sport and sending a clear message against gambling-related infractions.

3. Impact on Legacy: The debate often revolves around whether Rose's on-field accomplishments should be considered separately from his off-field actions. Some believe that his contributions to the game

merit recognition, while others assert that the ban is a crucial aspect of his legacy.

4. Hall of Fame Controversy: The question of whether Pete Rose should be eligible for induction into the Baseball Hall of Fame is a significant point of contention. The Hall of Fame's eligibility rules, which exclude individuals on MLB's permanently ineligible list, have been a source of debate.

5. Rehabilitation Efforts: Supporters of Rose often point to his efforts at rehabilitation, including public apologies, admissions of wrongdoing, and

community engagement, as signs of genuine remorse and a desire for redemption.

6. Perception of Fairness: Public opinion is also influenced by perceptions of fairness in the enforcement of rules and the consistency of disciplinary actions in professional sports. Some argue that Rose has served a long enough penalty, while others contend that maintaining the ban is crucial for the credibility of the league's rule

6.1 Reconciliation Efforts

Pete Rose has made various efforts toward reconciliation, seeking a resolution with Major League Baseball (MLB) and aiming to improve his public image. Some notable aspects of his reconciliation efforts include:

1. Admission of Wrongdoing (2004): In his 2004 autobiography, "My Prison Without Bars," Pete Rose admitted to betting on baseball, including games involving the Cincinnati Reds. This admission marked a significant step in acknowledging his actions and was seen by some as a form of accountability.

2. Public Apologies: Rose has publicly apologized on multiple occasions for his involvement in gambling activities and the impact it had on baseball. These apologies were aimed at fans, the baseball community, and anyone affected by his actions.

3. Reinstatement Appeals: Over the years, Rose has submitted formal requests for reinstatement to MLB. His appeals have included expressions of remorse and arguments that he has served a sufficient penalty for his actions. However, MLB

has maintained its decision to uphold the lifetime ban.

4. Community Engagement: Rose has engaged in community and charity activities, possibly as a way to demonstrate his commitment to positive contributions beyond the controversies of his past.

5. Public Relations Efforts: Rose has been involved in public relations efforts to improve his image, including media appearances and interviews where he discussed his past, his remorse, and his desire for a second chance.

6. Advocacy for Hall of Fame Eligibility: Rose and his supporters have advocated for his eligibility for induction into the Baseball Hall of Fame. They argue that his on-field achievements, including being the all-time hits leader, should be considered separate from his off-field transgressions. It's important to note that as of my last update, these efforts had not led to Pete Rose's reinstatement into MLB or his eligibility for the Hall of Fame.

6.2 Legacy

Pete Rose's legacy is multifaceted and reflects both his remarkable on-field achievements and the controversies surrounding his off-field actions. Here are key aspects of Pete Rose's legacy:

1. On-Field Achievements: Rose is celebrated as one of the greatest hitters in the history of baseball. He holds the record for hits in Major League Baseball (MLB), with 4,256 hits over his career. Rose's playing style, characterized by intensity and hustle, earned him the nickname "Charlie Hustle."

2. Versatility : Rose's versatility on the field is another hallmark of his legacy. He played multiple positions, including first base, outfield, and third base, showcasing his adaptability. His durability is evident in his long and productive career, spanning over 24 seasons.

3. Multiple All-Star Appearances: Rose was a 17-time All-Star, reflecting his consistent excellence and contributions to the sport. He played in 17 All-Star Games at five different positions.

4. Championships and MVP Awards: Rose played a key role in leading the Cincinnati

Reds to multiple championships, including World Series victories in 1975 and 1976. He was also awarded the Most Valuable Player (MVP) in the National League in 1973.

5. Banned from Baseball: Rose's legacy is overshadowed by the lifetime ban imposed by MLB in 1989. The ban resulted from allegations that he bet on baseball games, including those involving his team. This has prevented him from being considered for induction into the Hall of Fame.

6. Reconciliation Efforts: Despite the ban, Rose has made efforts to reconcile with

the baseball community and seek reinstatement. His admissions of wrongdoing, public apologies, and appeals for reinstatement have been part of this ongoing process.

7. Controversial Figures: Rose's legacy is emblematic of the complex relationship between sports, ethics, and personal conduct. While he remains a revered figure for his on-field achievements, the gambling controversy has left a lasting impact on how he is remembered in the broader context of baseball history.

8. Iconic Status: Despite the controversies, Pete Rose's impact on the game and his iconic status endure. His contributions to baseball, both positive and negative, continue to be a subject of discussion and debate among fans, analysts, and the broader baseball community.

6.3. Impact

Pete Rose's impact on baseball is profound and encompasses various aspects, both positive and negative:

1. All-Time Hits Leader: Rose's most significant on-field impact is his record as

MLB's all-time hits leader with 4,256 hits. His consistent ability to make contact and contribute offensively remains a benchmark in baseball history.

2. Versatility: Rose's versatility on the field is noteworthy. He played multiple positions, showcasing his adaptability and contributing to the success of his teams in different roles.

3. Competitive Spirit: Known for his intense work ethic and competitive spirit, Rose earned the nickname "Charlie Hustle." His approach to the game and

commitment to giving his best effort on every play left a lasting impression.

4. Championships and Awards: Rose played a pivotal role in leading the Cincinnati Reds to two World Series championships in 1975 and 1976. His contributions earned him accolades, including the National League MVP award in 1973.

5. Impact on Teammates: Rose's leadership and team-oriented mindset had a positive impact on his teammates. His dedication to the game set an example for those around him.

6. Controversial Legacy: The betting scandal and subsequent lifetime ban have significantly shaped Rose's legacy. The controversy surrounding his gambling activities and the ban have led to ongoing discussions about the intersection of personal conduct and the integrity of the sport.

7. Hall of Fame Exclusion: Despite his on-field achievements, Rose's impact is also marked by his exclusion from the Baseball Hall of Fame. The ban prevents him from being officially recognized among the game's all-time greats.

8. Ongoing Relevance: Pete Rose's impact endures as his name continues to be a point of discussion in the baseball community. The debate over his legacy reflects broader conversations about forgiveness, redemption, and the relationship between personal actions and professional recognition.

In summary, Pete Rose's impact is a complex mix of on-field excellence, versatility, leadership, and the enduring controversy surrounding his ban from baseball. His legacy remains a subject of fascination and debate within the broader context of baseball history.

6.4 Ongoing Influence On Baseball

January 2022, Pete Rose's ongoing influence on baseball primarily stems from the continued discussions and debates surrounding his legacy rather than active involvement in the sport. Here are key points:

1. Debate and Discussion: Rose's name remains a prominent topic of debate within the baseball community and among fans. Conversations often revolve around his ban, the impact on his legacy, and whether

he should be reinstated into baseball or considered for the Hall of Fame.

2. Legacy and Ethics Discussions: The ongoing influence lies in the broader conversations about the intersection of ethics, personal conduct, and the integrity of the game. Rose's case is frequently cited when discussing the consequences of gambling-related infractions in professional sports.

3. Hall of Fame Eligibility Debate: Rose's exclusion from the Hall of Fame continues to be a subject of discussion. The question of whether his on-field achievements

should outweigh his off-field actions remains unresolved, and his case is often referenced in discussions about Hall of Fame eligibility criteria.

4. Relevance in Betting Discussions: In discussions about sports betting and its impact on the integrity of professional sports, Pete Rose's case is frequently brought up as a historical example. His ban serves as a cautionary tale regarding the potential consequences for players, coaches, or officials involved in gambling activities.

5. Public Opinion and Perception: Rose's ongoing influence is also evident in the varying public opinions surrounding his legacy. Supporters advocate for forgiveness and reinstatement, while others emphasize the importance of upholding the rules and maintaining the integrity of the sport

CHAPTER 7: HIT RECORD

Pete Rose holds the record for the most hits in Major League Baseball (MLB) history. He achieved this milestone during his illustrious playing career. Here are some key details about Pete Rose's hit record:

1. Total Hits: Pete Rose recorded a total of 4,256 hits over the course of his MLB career. This accomplishment occurred over 24 seasons, during which he played for the Cincinnati Reds,

Philadelphia Phillies, and Montreal Expos.

.2. Hit Record Date: Rose surpassed the previous record held by Ty Cobb on September 11, 1985, at Riverfront Stadium in Cincinnati. He collected hit number 4,192, surpassing Cobb's longstanding record.

3. Consistency and Longevity: Rose's achievement reflects not only his exceptional hitting ability but also his remarkable consistency and longevity in the sport. His record remains a testament to his durability and skill as a contact hitter.

4. Charlie Hustle: Known for his nickname "Charlie Hustle," Rose was celebrated for his tenacious and hardworking approach to the game. His hustle and dedication contributed to his success on the field.

Despite this historic achievement, Pete Rose's legacy is complicated by his ban from baseball in 1989 due to allegations of betting on games, including those involving his team. This ban has prevented him from being considered for induction into the Baseball Hall of Fame. Please note that developments or changes in Pete Rose's situation beyond January 2022 would need to be checked for the latest information.

7.1. Statistical Legacy

Pete Rose's statistical legacy in baseball is marked by several remarkable achievements, reflecting his excellence on the field over a long and illustrious career. Here are key statistical aspects of Pete Rose's legacy:

1. All-Time Hits Leader: Rose's most prominent statistical accomplishment is his status as MLB's all-time hits leader. He

amassed a total of 4,256 hits during his career, surpassing the previous record held by Ty Cobb.

2. Longevity and Games Played: Rose's career longevity is reflected in his 24 seasons in the major leagues. He played in a record 3,562 games, showcasing both his endurance and consistent presence in lineups over the years.

3. Versatility and Positions Played: Rose's versatility is evident in the fact that he played multiple positions during his career, including first base, outfield, and

third base. This adaptability contributed to his overall impact on the game.

4. Batting Average and On-Base Percentage: Rose consistently maintained a high batting average throughout his career. His lifetime batting average is .303, and he had an on-base percentage of .375, emphasizing his ability to reach base consistently.

5. Runs Scored: Rose scored a significant number of runs over his career, crossing the plate 2,165 times. His ability to contribute both with hits and runs showcases his offensive impact.

6. Hit Streaks: Rose had multiple impressive hit streaks during his career, including a 44-game hit streak in 1978, which stands as the second-longest in MLB history.

7. Accolades and Awards: Rose earned numerous accolades and awards, including 17 All-Star selections, three batting titles, and the National League MVP award in 1973. These accomplishments contribute to his statistical legacy.

While Rose's on-field statistics solidify his place as one of the greatest hitters in baseball history, his statistical legacy is complicated by his ban from baseball in 1989 due to gambling-related allegations. This ban has prevented him from being eligible for induction into the Baseball Hall of Fame.

CHAPTER 8: LIFE AFTER THE GAME

Pete Rose's life after his playing career has been marked by various activities, including business ventures, public appearances, and continued involvement in the world of baseball. Here are some aspects of Pete Rose's life after the game:

1. Managing Career: After retiring as a player, Pete Rose transitioned to a career as a manager. He managed the Cincinnati Reds from 1984 to 1989, leading the team to a World Series title in 1990. However,

his managerial career ended abruptly due to his ban from baseball in 1989.

2. Business Ventures: Rose has been involved in various business ventures, including owning and operating sports memorabilia stores. His autograph signings and appearances at sports collectible events have been a source of income and engagement with fans.

3. Broadcasting and Media: Rose has worked as a baseball analyst for various media outlets, providing commentary and analysis on the sport. His insights into the game have been sought after, contributing

to his continued presence in the public eye.

4. Public Appearances : Rose has made public appearances at events, autograph signings, and promotional activities. Despite his ban from baseball, he remains a popular figure among fans who seek his autograph and engage with him at events.

5. Books and Autobiography: Pete Rose has authored several books, including his autobiography titled "My Prison Without Bars," which was published in 2004. In the book, he candidly discussed his life,

playing career, and the controversies surrounding his ban from baseball.

6. Reinstatement Efforts: Rose has persistently sought reinstatement into baseball, making formal appeals to MLB commissioners. Despite repeated denials, he has continued to express a desire for reconciliation with the sport and a chance to contribute to the game.

7. Personal Challenges: Rose has faced personal challenges, including legal issues. In addition to the defamation lawsuit he filed against John Dowd (which was settled out of court), he has encountered

legal troubles unrelated to baseball, including tax evasion charges.

8.1. Public Image and Legacy

Pete Rose's public image and legacy remain complex due to the controversies surrounding his gambling activities. His ongoing efforts for reinstatement and public appearances contribute to the ongoing discussions about his place in baseball history.

It's important to note that developments in Pete Rose's life after the game may have occurred since my last knowledge update in January 2022. For the latest

information, checking more recent sources
is recommended.

has been marked by various activities,
including business ventures, public
appearances, and continued involvement
in the world of baseball. Here are some
aspects of Pete Rose's life after the game:

1. Managing Career: After retiring as a
player, Pete Rose transitioned to a career
as a manager. He managed the Cincinnati
Reds from 1984 to 1989, leading the team
to a World Series title in 1990. However,
his managerial career ended abruptly due
to his ban from baseball in 1989.

2. Business Ventures: Rose has been involved in various business ventures, including owning and operating sports memorabilia stores. His autograph signings and appearances at sports collectible events have been a source of income and engagement with fans.

3. Broadcasting and Media: Rose has worked as a baseball analyst for various media outlets, providing commentary and analysis on the sport. His insights into the game have been sought after, contributing to his continued presence in the public eye.

4. Public Appearances and Autograph Signings: Rose has made public appearances at events, autograph signings, and promotional activities. Despite his ban from baseball, he remains a popular figure among fans who seek his autograph and engage with him at events.

Books and Autobiography: Pete Rose has authored several books, including his autobiography titled "My Prison Without Bars," which was published in 2004. In the book, he candidly discussed his life, playing career, and the controversies surrounding his ban from baseball.

5. Reinstatement Efforts: Rose has persistently sought reinstatement into baseball, making formal appeals to MLB commissioners. Despite repeated denials, he has continued to express a desire for reconciliation with the sport and a chance to contribute to the game.

6. Personal Challenges: Rose has faced personal challenges, including legal issues. In addition to the defamation lawsuit he filed against John Dowd (which was settled out of court), he has encountered legal troubles unrelated to baseball, including tax evasion charges.

7. Public Image and Legacy: Pete Rose's public image and legacy remain complex due to the controversies surrounding his gambling activities. His ongoing efforts for reinstatement and public appearances contribute to the ongoing discussions about his place in baseball history.

It's important to note that developments in Pete Rose's life after the game may have occurred since my last knowledge update in January 2022.

8.2. Beyond The Diamond – A Playbook For Entrepreneurial Success"

In this comprehensive exploration of Pete Rose's entrepreneurial ventures, we delve into the multifaceted career of the baseball legend beyond the realm of the diamond. Pete Rose, widely known as "Charlie Hustle" for his relentless work ethic on the baseball field, demonstrated a similar determination and entrepreneurial spirit in various business endeavors. The book navigates through Rose's transition from a stellar baseball career to a shrewd entrepreneur, showcasing the strategic moves and calculated risks he took to establish himself in the business world. From endorsements and memorabilia to owning and operating his own sports bar, Pete Rose leveraged his iconic status to build a brand that extended far beyond the confines of the baseball stadium.

Readers will gain insights into the challenges Rose faced, including controversies that paralleled his entrepreneurial journey. The book explores how Rose navigated through legal issues and public scrutiny, offering a candid look at the highs and lows of his business ventures.

Additionally, "Pete Rose: Beyond the Diamond" sheds light on Rose's involvement in sports betting and the subsequent ban from baseball. The narrative doesn't shy away from the controversies surrounding his choices, providing a balanced perspective on how these events impacted both his baseball legacy and entrepreneurial endeavors. Through interviews with business associates, industry experts, and Rose himself, this book offers a nuanced and detailed portrait of Pete Rose as an entrepreneur. It's a compelling narrative that goes beyond the statistics of his baseball career, illustrating how his resilience, determination, and business acumen shaped a legacy that extends far beyond the confines of the baseball diamond.

8.3. Beyond Baseball

This insightful exploration uncovers the layers of Pete Rose's life beyond the diamond, delving into the personal, professional, and controversial aspects that have defined his legacy. From his early days on the sandlots of Cincinnati to becoming one of baseball's all-time greats, the book provides a nuanced portrait of Rose's journey.

Readers will discover the man behind the iconic "Charlie Hustle" persona, exploring Rose's family life, relationships, and the pivotal moments that shaped him both on and off the field. The narrative goes beyond the statistics, offering a glimpse into the challenges and triumphs that marked Rose's path to greatness.

The book also addresses the controversies that have surrounded Rose, including his ban from baseball due to allegations of sports betting. By examining these events in the broader context of his life, "Pete Rose: Beyond Baseball" seeks to provide a comprehensive understanding of the complexities that define this legendary figure.

Furthermore, the exploration extends to Rose's post-baseball endeavors, showcasing his entrepreneurial ventures, community involvement, and the enduring impact he has had beyond the realm of sports. Through interviews, anecdotes, and a thorough examination of historical records, this book paints a vivid picture of Pete Rose's enduring legacy as a person, player, and public figure.

8.4. Public Appearances :Beyond The Spotlight

This detailed examination offers readers an in-depth perspective on Pete Rose's public appearances, unraveling the various dimensions of his engagements beyond the baseball field. From autograph signings and speaking engagements to public events and appearances, the book navigates through the public sphere where Rose has continued to captivate audiences. Readers will gain insights into the dynamics of Rose's interactions with fans, media, and the public at large. The narrative explores the impact of his celebrity status on these appearances, shedding light on how Rose's persona has evolved in the public eye.

The book also addresses the challenges and controversies that have accompanied Rose's public life, including the ongoing dialogue surrounding his ban from baseball and its influence on his public image. Through a series of interviews, firsthand accounts, and a meticulous examination of public records, this book provides a comprehensive overview of Pete Rose's presence in the public domain. Whether it's on the stage at a baseball event, signing autographs at a memorabilia show, or engaging with fans through various platforms, "Pete Rose: Beyond the

Spotlight" captures the essence of Rose's public appearances, offering readers a nuanced understanding of the man behind the iconic figure.

8.5. Media Presence

This insightful exploration delves into the intricate tapestry of Pete Rose's media presence, offering readers a comprehensive look at how he has been portrayed and perceived through various forms of media. From newspaper headlines and television interviews to social media and beyond, the book unravels the layers of Rose's relationship with the media.

Readers will gain insights into how Rose's image has been shaped, challenged, and transformed over the years, examining the role of media in both celebrating his baseball achievements and scrutinizing his personal and professional choices. The narrative explores the highs and lows of Rose's media coverage, from the exhilaration of record-breaking moments to the controversies that have cast a shadow on his legacy.

The book also addresses Rose's engagement with media, including interviews, public statements, and his use of social platforms. It delves into how he has navigated the challenges posed by the media landscape, particularly in the context of his ban from baseball and other controversies.

Through a meticulous analysis of news articles, broadcast segments, and social media interactions, "Pete Rose: Beyond the Headlines" provides a nuanced understanding of the complex interplay between Pete Rose and the media. This exploration goes beyond the surface to uncover the impact of media on shaping public perception and the enduring legacy of a figure who has remained a focal point in the media landscape for decades.

CHAPER 9: A TIMELESS LEGACY IN BASEBALL HISTORY

This compelling exploration delves into the enduring presence of Pete Rose in the annals of baseball history, showcasing how his impact transcends eras and continues to shape the narrative of America's pastime.

The book navigates through Rose's unparalleled achievements on the field, including his record-breaking hits and the tenacious "Charlie Hustle" approach that made him a baseball icon. It meticulously examines the statistical milestones that cemented Rose's place in history and analyzes his contributions to the evolution of the game.

Beyond the statistics, the narrative explores Rose's complex legacy, addressing the controversies that have marked his career. From the highs of World Series victories to the lows of the ban from baseball, readers gain a nuanced understanding of the multifaceted nature of Rose's enduring presence.

The book also delves into Rose's impact off the field, including his roles as a manager, broadcaster, and ambassador for the sport. Through interviews, anecdotes, and historical context, it highlights how Rose's influence extends beyond his playing days, leaving an indelible mark on the sport he dedicated his life to "Pete Rose: A Timeless Legacy in Baseball History" is a comprehensive examination of a figure who remains a central character in the ongoing narrative of baseball, illustrating how his legacy persists, evolves, and contributes to the rich tapestry of the sport's history

CONCLUSION

In the tale of Pete Rose, we witness the complexities of a baseball icon's journey – a rise marked by unparalleled prowess, a fall tainted by controversy. Yet, amidst the shadows, Rose leaves an indelible legacy, reminding us that the man, the myth, and the legend are woven into the fabric of the sport, creating a narrative that is as unforgettable as it is controversial. His story serves as a testament to the enduring impact of both triumphs and tribulations on the enduring spirit of baseball

Pete Rose, a baseball icon, encapsulates a saga of unparalleled prowess, the rise to glory, and a precipitous fall marked by controversy. Beyond the statistics and achievements lies the man, the myth, and the legend, whose indomitable spirit and passion for the game are eternally etched in the annals of baseball history. Despite the shadows cast by his transgressions, Rose's legacy is unforgettable, serving as a poignant reminder that greatness and imperfection coexist in the complex tapestry of sports. His story is not just a chronicle of triumphs and pitfalls but a reflection of the enduring human drama that defines the essence of baseball, making Pete Rose an enduring figure in the hearts of fans, leaving an indelible mark on the sport he both elevated and complicated.